30-Day Prayer Journal

PRAYER JOURNAL FOR BREAST CANCER WARRIORS, THRIVERS, & SURVIVORS

Michelle Williford

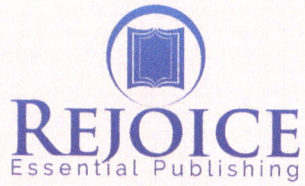

Copyright © 2024 by **Michelle Williford**

All rights reserved. No part of this publication may be reproduced, distributed or transmitted in any form or by any means, including photocopying, recording, or other electronic or mechanical methods, without the prior written permission of the publisher, except in the case of brief quotations embodied in critical reviews and certain other noncommercial uses permit-ted by copyright law. For mission requests, write to the publisher, addressed " Attention: Permissions Coordinator," at the address below.

Michelle Williford /Rejoice Essential Publishing

PO BOX 512

Effingham, SC 29541

www.republishing.org

Author's Contact:

www.sheshinez.org

Unless otherwise indicated, scripture is taken from the King James Version.

30-Day Prayer Journal/ Michelle Williford

Healing Journal

HEALING IS A BLESSING THAT BELONGS TO EVERY CHILD OF GOD. IT IS YOUR BLOOD-BOUGHT RIGHT TO LIVE IN GOOD HEALTH EVERY DAY OF YOUR LIFE SIMPLY BECAUSE YOU BELONG TO THE FAMILY OF GOD. JESUS PAID THE ULTIMATE PRICE FOR YOU TO BE HEALED, BOTH PHYSICALLY AND SPIRITUALLY. IT BRINGS HIM GREAT GLORY WHEN WE CHOOSE TO LIVE THE LIFE OF HEALTH AND WHOLENESS THAT HE PURCHASED FOR US ON THE CROSS. EMBRACE THIS GIFT OF HEALING WITH GRATITUDE AND FAITH, KNOWING THAT GOD'S DESIRE IS FOR YOU TO EXPERIENCE ABUNDANT LIFE IN EVERY WAY, INCLUDING YOUR HEALTH. TRUST IN HIS LOVE AND PROVISION, AND WALK IN THE TRUTH THAT YOU ARE A BELOVED CHILD OF GOD, DESERVING OF HIS HEALING TOUCH.

THIS 30-DAY PRAYER JOURNAL IS TO HELP REMIND YOU OF THE HEALING THAT IS RIGHTFULLY YOURS! START YOUR DAY OFF PRAYING THE SCRIPTURES. WRITE WHAT IS IN YOUR HEART AND WHAT GOD IS SPEAKING TO YOU IN THAT MOMENT. REMEMBER THE PRAYERS HE HAS ALREADY ANSWERED, AND READ THE PROMPTS ON THE VISUAL JOURNAL AND RESPOND IN EACH SECTION.

Just Breathe - Day 1

CAST ALL YOUR ANXIETY ON HIM BECAUSE HE CARES FOR YOU.
1 PETER 5: 7

Cancer can be a scary word, but it doesn't have to be. Now is the time to cast that fear over to God. Trust in His plan and find comfort in knowing that you are never alone in this battle.

Through prayer, trust, and belief, you can find the strength to face each day with courage and hope. Remember that you are surrounded by love and support, and you have the power to overcome any challenges that come your way. Stay positive, keep fighting, and believe that you will get through this. Tell God how you feel today and be honest about it.......

_____
_____
_____
_____
_____
_____
_____
_____
_____
_____
_____
_____
_____
_____

Visual Journal

Date: _____

Read the prompts below and respond by filling each space provided with images and words that come into mind.

When I woke up this morning, I felt.....	Things I wish I can change about today:

I am proud of myself today because...	What I prayed for today....

He is with you! Day 2

"FEAR NOT, FOR I AM WITH YOU; BE NOT DISMAYED, FOR I AM YOUR GOD. I WILL STRENGTHEN YOU, YES, I WILL HELP YOU, I WILL UPHOLD YOU WITH MY RIGHTEOUS RIGHT HAND." ISAIAH 41: 10

In this journey ahead, you will not have to walk alone. Yes, there will be moments when it all feels like too much to bear - the countless doctor visits, the daunting surgeries - but remember, you are never alone. He will be there to guide you, to provide you with the strength you need, and to lift you up when you feel like you can't go on. Through the highs and lows, He will be by your side, giving you the courage to face whatever challenges come your way. So take each step with faith, knowing that you are never alone in this journey.

Knowing that God is with you, list the names of your support team below. Having a support team you can depend on, helps you along your journey. Remember to pray over your support team.

_____
_____
_____
_____
_____
_____
_____
_____

Visual Journal

Date: _____

Read the prompts below and respond by filling each space provided with images and words that come into mind.

When I woke up this morning, I felt.....	Things I wish I can change about today:
I am proud of myself today because...	What I prayed for today....

The Peace of God - Day 3

DO NOT BE ANXIOUS ABOUT ANYTHING, BUT IN EVERY SITUATION, BY PRAYER AND PETITION, WITH THANKSGIVING, PRESENT YOUR REQUESTS TO GOD. AND THE PEACE OF GOD, WHICH TRANSCENDS ALL UNDERSTANDING, WILL GUARD YOUR HEARTS AND YOUR MINDS IN CHRIST JESUS.
PHILIPPIANS 4: 6-7

Revealing your diagnosis to your family can be a daunting and anxiety-inducing task. It's essential to seek guidance through prayer and connect with God on who to confide in about your condition. Guarding your heart against negative cancer outcomes is crucial for maintaining your peace of mind. Instead of focusing on worst-case scenarios, allow the peace of God to envelop you and provide comfort during this challenging time. Trust in His guidance and find solace in knowing that you are not alone in this journey.
Stay strong and remember that you are surrounded by love and support, both from your family and from The Most High God.
What is your prayer today?

_____
_____
_____
_____
_____
_____
_____
_____

Visual Journal

Date: _____

Read the prompts below and respond by filling each space provided with images and words that come into mind.

When I woke up this morning, I felt.....	Things I wish I can change about today:
I am proud of myself today because...	What I prayed for today....

Forgiveness - Day 4

AND WHENEVER YOU STAND PRAYING, IF YOU HAVE ANYTHING AGAINST ANYONE, FORGIVE HIM, THAT YOUR FATHER IN HEAVEN MAY ALSO FORGIVE YOU YOUR TRESPASSES.
MARK 11: 25

Forgiveness is essential to healing. Unforgiveness in our hearts hinders our faith from working. The Father can't forgive us if we haven't forgiven others.

Think of all the people who have hurt you or caused you harm and decide today that you forgive them for their offenses against you. List their names below and pray for them.

_____
_____
_____
_____
_____
_____
_____
_____
_____
_____
_____
_____

Visual Journal

Date: _____

Read the prompts below and respond by filling each space provided with images and words that come into mind.

When I woke up this morning, I felt.....	Things I wish I can change about today:
I am proud of myself today because...	What I prayed for today....

Your Faith – Day 5

HE SAID TO HER, " DAUGHTER, YOUR FAITH HAS HEALED YOU. GO IN PEACE AND BE FREED FROM YOUR SUFFERING."
MARK 5: 34

How is your faith today? The Bible says that faith comes by hearing, and hearing the Word of God (Romans 10:7)

Healing is your portion. All you need is Faith! When Jesus died on the cross, He shed his blood for the remission of our sins, His body was wounded for our transgressions and by his stripes we were HEALED. This means that if you have accepted Jesus as Lord and Savior of your life, when you got SAVED, you did not just receive forgiveness of your SINS but also healing for your BODY.
Tell God what you are believing Him for:

_____
_____
_____
_____
_____
_____
_____
_____

Visual Journal

Date: _____

Read the prompts below and respond by filling each space provided with images and words that come into mind.

When I woke up this morning, I felt.....	Things I wish I can change about today:
I am proud of myself today because...	What I prayed for today....

His Benefits - Day 6

BLESS THE LORD, O MY SOUL, AND FORGET NOT ALL HIS BENEFITS; WHO FORGIVES ALL YOUR INIQUITIES; WHO HEALS ALL YOUR DISEASES.
PSALM 103: 2-3

Despite what the doctors have said, command your soul to praise the Lord! Bless the Lord with all your heart and all your soul! There are benefits in praising the Lord, even when your body does not feel like it.

When you choose to lift your spirit in praise, you invite positivity and hope into your life. Praise has the power to uplift your soul and bring peace to your mind, regardless of the circumstances. So, in moments of doubt or despair, remember to turn to the Lord in praise, for He is the source of strength and comfort. Trust in His goodness and let your praises be a beacon of light in the darkness.

What are you praising God for today?

_____
_____
_____
_____
_____
_____
_____

Visual Journal

Date: _____

Read the prompts below and respond by filling each space provided with images and words that come into mind.

| When I woke up this morning, I felt..... | Things I wish I can change about today: |

| I am proud of myself today because... | What I prayed for today.... |

Prosper – Day 7

BELOVED, I PRAY THAT YOU MAY PROSPER IN ALL THINGS AND BE IN HEALTH, JUST AS YOUR SOUL PROSPERS.
3 JOHN 1: 2

God calls you His Beloved. Beloved is defined as "dearly loved". This means that you are cherished and valued by the Creator of the universe. God wants us to prosper in every area of our lives, including our health. By embracing our identity as God's Beloved, we can walk in abundance and fulfillment. Let us remember that we are deeply loved and that God desires good things for us. With this awareness, we can trust in His plans for our well-being and trust that He will guide us toward a life of prosperity and wholeness. Let us embrace our identity as Beloved and walk in the fullness of God's love and blessings.

Take this time to take inventory of your life. What areas of your life need to prosper? What areas will you believe God to prosper? List them below and pray over them.

_____
_____
_____
_____
_____
_____
_____
_____

Visual Journal

Date: _____

Read the prompts below and respond by filling each space provided with images and words that come into mind.

When I woke up this morning, I felt.....	Things I wish I can change about today:
I am proud of myself today because...	What I prayed for today....

Your Prayer Circle - Day 8

IS ANYONE AMONG YOU SICK? LET THEM CALL THE ELDERS OF THE CHURCH TO PRAY OVER THEM AND ANOINT THEM WITH OIL IN THE NAME OF THE LORD. AND THE PRAYER OFFERED IN FAITH WILL MAKE THE SICK PERSON WELL; THE LORD WILL RAISE THEM UP. IF THEY HAVE SINNED, THEY WILL BE FORGIVEN. THEREFORE CONFESS YOUR SINS TO EACH OTHER AND PRAY FOR EACH OTHER SO THAT YOU MAY BE HEALED. THE PRAYER OF A RIGHTEOUS PERSON IS POWERFUL AND EFFECTIVE

JAMES 5: 14-16

Who is in your prayer circle? It is crucial to involve your church community or someone you trust, who is strong in their faith, to join you in prayer. Take time to pray and seek guidance from the Lord on who should be part of your prayer circle. Make a list of their names and lift them up in prayer as well. By surrounding yourself with individuals who are committed to praying for you, you can find strength and support during challenging times. Remember, you are not alone in your journey, and your faith community is there to offer their prayers and support. Trust in the power of collective prayer to uplift and sustain you. List their names and pray over them.

_____
_____
_____
_____
_____
_____
_____

Visual Journal

Date: _____

Read the prompts below and respond by filling each space provided with images and words that come into mind.

When I woke up this morning, I felt.....	Things I wish I can change about today:
I am proud of myself today because...	What I prayed for today....

By His Stripes...Day 9

SURELY HE HATH BORNE OUR GRIEFS AND CARRIED OUR SORROWS; YET WE DID ESTEEM HIM STRICKEN, SMITTEN OF GOD, AND AFFLICTED. BUT HE WAS WOUNDED FOR OUR TRANSGRESSIONS; HE WAS BRUISED FOR OUR INIQUITIES. THE CHASTISEMENT OF OUR PEACE WAS UPON HIM, AND WITH HIS STRIPES WE ARE HEALED.
ISAIAH 53: 4-5

    The Bible says, by His stripes, we are healed (Isaiah 53:5). The words "we are healed" are in past tense and means that our healing has been fully secured on the cross by Christ over 2,000 years ago. This powerful statement embodies the promise of redemption and restoration for all who believe. "By His Stripes We Are Healed" reminds us of the profound sacrifice that Christ made for our eternal well-being. It signifies not only physical healing but also emotional, spiritual, and mental wholeness. In embracing this truth, we acknowledge that Christ's love transcends our pain and brokenness, offering us a new beginning and a renewed sense of hope. Who else do you know that needs healing? List their names and pray over them.

_____
_____
_____
_____
_____
_____
_____
_____
_____

Visual Journal

Date: _____

Read the prompts below and respond by filling each space provided with images and words that come into mind.

When I woke up this morning, I felt.....

Things I wish I can change about today:

I am proud of myself today because...

What I prayed for today....

Restoration – Day 10

BUT I WILL RESTORE YOU TO HEALTH AND HEAL YOUR WOUNDS,' DECLARES THE LORD, JEREMIAH 30: 17

In the Bible, restoration is always in abundance. When something is restored, it is always better than it was to begin with. So, rejoice in advance for the restoration of your health! Trust that the healing process will surpass your expectations and bring about a renewed sense of well-being. Just like a broken vessel being meticulously pieced back together into a masterpiece, your health will be restored to a level of wholeness that is truly extraordinary. Remember the promise in Psalm 91 that He will satisfy you with long life, embracing each day with gratitude and optimism for the blessings that lie ahead. Trust in the divine plan for your health and well-being, knowing that you are truly cherished and cared for beyond measure. Remember this promise!

_____
_____
_____
_____
_____
_____
_____
_____

Visual Journal

Date: _____

Read the prompts below and respond by filling each space provided with images and words that come into mind.

When I woke up this morning, I felt.....

Things I wish I can change about today:

I am proud of myself today because...

What I prayed for today....

Abundant Peace - Day 11

NEVERTHELESS, I WILL BRING HEALTH AND HEALING TO IT; I WILL HEAL MY PEOPLE AND WILL LET THEM ENJOY ABUNDANT PEACE AND SECURITY.
JEREMIAH 33: 6

After the healing, comes abundant peace and security. Lord, thank You for revealing an abundance of Your truth, peace, and security in my life. I receive my healing and I will walk in divine health, in Jesus' name, so be it!
In the midst of chaos and uncertainty, I find comfort in Your promises and strength in Your presence. May Your peace that surpasses all understanding guard my heart and mind, keeping me grounded in Your love and protection. With each step I take, I am guided by Your light, knowing that You are my refuge and strength. Grant me the wisdom to trust in Your plan and the courage to walk in faith, knowing that You hold my future in Your hands. Thank You, Lord, for your grace and mercy that sustain me through every trial and tribulation. Amen.
Think of another time when God gave you peace about the matter.

_____
_____
_____
_____
_____
_____
_____
_____

Visual Journal

Date: _____

Read the prompts below and respond by filling each space provided with images and words that come into mind.

When I woke up this morning, I felt.....	Things I wish I can change about today:

I am proud of myself today because...	What I prayed for today....

All Needs - Day 12

AND MY GOD WILL MEET ALL YOUR NEEDS ACCORDING TO THE RICHES OF HIS GLORY IN CHRIST JESUS.
PHILIPPIANS 4:19

God knows our daily needs even before we utter a word. When we trust Him to provide for us, our faith blossoms and we mature spiritually. By turning to God with our requests and wholeheartedly believing in His power, we open the door for Him to fulfill all our needs - whether they be spiritual enlightenment or physical sustenance. God is always ready to listen to our prayers and offer His divine support. All we have to do is approach Him with sincerity and have faith that He will guide us through all walks of life. Trust in God's providence, and you will witness miracles unfold before your very eyes. Make a list of all the times that God supplied a need in your life and meditate on them.

_____
_____
_____
_____
_____
_____
_____
_____

Visual Journal

Date: _____

Read the prompts below and respond by filling each space provided with images and words that come into mind.

When I woke up this morning, I felt.....

Things I wish I can change about today:

I am proud of myself today because...

What I prayed for today....

Good Medicine - Day 13

A CHEERFUL HEART IS GOOD MEDICINE, BUT A CRUSHED SPIRIT DRIES UP THE BONES
PROVERBS 17:22

God created us in such a beautiful way that joy and humor are meant to be an intricate part of our lives. The connection between our emotional health and physical health shows that when we have a positive outlook, we tend to have a positive outcome. It is important to cultivate a mindset that embraces laughter and finds joy in the smallest of things. Laughter is indeed the best medicine, boosting our immune system and reducing stress levels. When we approach life with a light heart and a sense of humor, we not only improve our own well-being but also brighten the world around us. Let us remember to sprinkle laughter and joy into our everyday lives, for it is through these simple pleasures that we find true happiness and fulfillment. What really made you laugh today?

_____
_____
_____
_____
_____
_____
_____

Visual Journal

Date: _____

Read the prompts below and respond by filling each space provided with images and words that come into mind.

When I woke up this morning, I felt.....	Things I wish I can change about today:
I am proud of myself today because...	What I prayed for today....

Strength - Day 14

LORD, BE GRACIOUS TO US; WE LONG FOR YOU.
BE OUR STRENGTH EVERY MORNING, OUR SALVATION IN TIME OF DISTRESS.
ISAIAH 33:2

Going through radiation, chemotherapy, and/or surgery can be challenging. It's important to remember to start your day with our Gracious Father, seeking strength and comfort in Him. Call out to God every morning, asking for His guidance and support as you navigate through the challenges that lie ahead. By committing each day to The Lord, you can find the peace and resilience you need to face whatever comes your way. Trust in His love and mercy to carry you through difficult times and know that you are never alone in your journey towards healing and recovery. Write down your appointment dates and remember to seek the Lord before going in for your visit.

_____
_____
_____
_____
_____
_____
_____

Visual Journal

Date: _____

Read the prompts below and respond by filling each space provided with images and words that come into mind.

When I woke up this morning, I felt.....

Things I wish I can change about today:

I am proud of myself today because...

What I prayed for today....

Lord Help Me - Day 15

LORD MY GOD, I CALLED TO YOU FOR HELP, AND YOU HEALED ME.
PSALM 3:2

We know that the promises of God are Yes and Amen for the believer. God is faithful to answer the cry of the believer. In moments of healing, remember to give God thanks for every time your body is restored and made whole. In times of medical procedures and challenges, remember to give Him praise after making it through each one, knowing that His grace and strength carried you. Let gratitude be your response, for God's faithfulness endures through every trial and triumph. Trust in His promises, for He is a God who keeps His word and sustains His people with unwavering love.

_____
_____
_____
_____
_____
_____
_____

Visual Journal

Date: _____

Read the prompts below and respond by filling each space provided with images and words that come into mind.

When I woke up this morning, I felt.....	Things I wish I can change about today:
I am proud of myself today because...	What I prayed for today....

Don't Give Up! - Day 16

HAVE MERCY ON ME, LORD, FOR I AM FAINT; HEAL ME, LORD, FOR MY BONES ARE IN AGONY.

PSALM 6:2

In the middle of your weakness, know that God is your strength and that He is gracious. God is good. God loves you and hears your cries. Even when it feels like the medicine is taking a toll on you, God is there, holding you in His loving embrace. Trust in His plan for you and have faith that He will guide you through the challenges you face. Remember that you are never alone, for God is always by your side, ready to comfort you and give you strength. In times of darkness, let the light of God's love shine upon you and illuminate your path. Embrace His grace and know that you are deeply cherished and cared for beyond measure. Keep going!

_____
_____
_____
_____
_____
_____
_____
_____

Visual Journal

Date: _____

Read the prompts below and respond by filling each space provided with images and words that come into mind.

When I woke up this morning, I felt.....	Things I wish I can change about today:
I am proud of myself today because...	What I prayed for today....

Just Believe! Day 17

HEARING THIS, JESUS SAID TO JAIRUS, " DON' T BE AFRAID; JUST BELIEVE, AND SHE WILL BE HEALED."
LUKE 8: 50

Jesus demonstrated his compassion and miraculous power when he willingly healed a woman who had been suffering from a serious medical issue for years. His ability to bring about physical healing is a testament to his divine nature and unwavering love for us. Moreover, Jesus showed that He has the power and the desire to perform even greater miracles, such as raising a dead girl back to life. These profound moments serve as a reminder that through faith and belief in Jesus, anything is possible. Trust in His infinite power and unwavering love, and miracles beyond imagination can come to fruition. Just believe in the miracles that Jesus can perform, and open your heart to receive his grace and blessings.

_____
_____
_____
_____
_____
_____
_____
_____

Visual Journal

Date: _____

Read the prompts below and respond by filling each space provided with images and words that come into mind.

When I woke up this morning, I felt.....

Things I wish I can change about today:

I am proud of myself today because...

What I prayed for today....

Rise Up With Healing – Day 18

BUT FOR YOU WHO REVERE MY NAME, THE SUN OF RIGHTEOUSNESS WILL RISE WITH HEALING IN ITS RAYS. AND YOU WILL GO OUT AND FROLIC LIKE WELL-FED CALVES. MALACHI 4: 2

Those who wholeheartedly worship the Lord with faith and devotion are promised complete healing and well-being. The healing power of the Lord will touch every soul, soothe wounds, and restore peace. Through the act of worship, individuals can connect with God and He can provide comfort and healing in times of need. Trusting in the Lord's divine guidance and mercy can lead to a transformation that touches not only the body but also the mind and spirit. The path to wholeness and wellness begins with a sincere heart and a steadfast commitment to praising and honoring the Lord, for it is through this dedication that true healing can be achieved.

_____
_____
_____
_____
_____
_____
_____
_____
_____

Visual Journal

Date: _____

Read the prompts below and respond by filling each space provided with images and words that come into mind.

When I woke up this morning, I felt.....	Things I wish I can change about today:
I am proud of myself today because...	What I prayed for today....

You Are The One I Praise! Day 19

HEAL ME, LORD, AND I WILL BE HEALED; SAVE ME AND I WILL BE SAVED, FOR YOU ARE THE ONE I PRAISE.
JEREMIAH 17: 14

"Heal me, Lord, and I will be healed; save me and I will be saved, for you are the one I praise." These words echo the deep longing for spiritual and physical restoration, acknowledging that true healing comes from God. In times of distress and difficulty, turning to God for strength can bring a sense of peace and hope. The act of surrendering and putting one's faith in the ultimate healer can provide comfort and reassurance in the face of adversity. Through prayer, one can find healing for the body, mind, and soul, trusting in the power of divine grace to bring wholeness and restoration.
Don't forget that God dwells in the praises! Release a sound of praise in your house today and every day!

_____
_____
_____
_____
_____
_____
_____
_____

Visual Journal

Date: _____

Read the prompts below and respond by filling each space provided with images and words that come into mind.

When I woke up this morning, I felt.....	Things I wish I can change about today:
I am proud of myself today because...	What I prayed for today....

Praises to The Most High God - Day 20

HE SENT OUT HIS WORD AND HEALED THEM; HE RESCUED THEM FROM THE GRAVE.
PSALM 107: 20

When you need physical healing, remember that God sends His Word to heal you. Keep crying out to Him, for He listens to your prayers. Cry out in faith, believing in His power to heal. Cry out with thanksgiving, grateful for His mercy and grace. And in the spirit of worship, trust that God's healing hand is upon you. Adore Him for His love and compassion, knowing that He is the ultimate healer. Keep your heart open to His guidance and take comfort in the knowledge that His healing touch is always near. Speak the Word of God over your life EVERYDAY!

_____
_____
_____
_____
_____
_____
_____

Visual Journal

Date: _____

Read the prompts below and respond by filling each space provided with images and words that come into mind.

When I woke up this morning, I felt.....	Things I wish I can change about today:
I am proud of myself today because...	What I prayed for today....

He Watches Over His Word – Day 21

THE LORD SAID TO ME, "YOU HAVE SEEN CORRECTLY, FOR I AM WATCHING TO SEE THAT MY WORD IS FULFILLED."
JEREMIAH 1: 12

The Spirit of God would always accompany the Word, ensuring that it would carry out the Lord's intended purpose. This divine partnership between the Word and the Spirit serves as a powerful assurance that God's will and plan will be fulfilled through the spoken or written Word. The presence of the Spirit guarantees that the Word will not return void but will achieve its desired outcome. Therefore, as we engage with the Word of God, let us be mindful of the vital role of the Spirit in bringing its truths to life and bringing about transformation and healing in our lives. Trust in the Word and the Spirit working together to bring about the fulfillment of God's purposes in and through us. I get excited every time I read this scripture because I know that God's Word will not return to him void and that we are HEALED!

_____
_____
_____
_____
_____
_____
_____
_____

Visual Journal

Date: _____

Read the prompts below and respond by filling each space provided with images and words that come into mind.

When I woke up this morning, I felt.....	Things I wish I can change about today:
I am proud of myself today because...	What I prayed for today....

Binding Up Wounds - Day 22

HE HEALS THE BROKENHEARTED AND BINDS UP THEIR WOUNDS.
PSALM 147: 3

The Psalmist beautifully portrays God as a compassionate Healer of the brokenhearted. In times of despair and shattered spirits, God is there to mend the wounds and bring comfort to those who are hurting. His love knows no bounds, and His healing touch can restore even the most broken souls. Through faith and prayer, one can find comfort in knowing that God is there to heal the broken pieces and mend the shattered hearts. It is a testament to the divine power of God's love and grace that He can bring healing and restoration to those who are in need.

_____
_____
_____
_____
_____
_____
_____
_____

Visual Journal

Date: _____

Read the prompts below and respond by filling each space provided with images and words that come into mind.

When I woke up this morning, I felt.....	Things I wish I can change about today:
I am proud of myself today because...	What I prayed for today....

God is Faithful – Day 23

THE LORD SUSTAINS THEM ON THEIR SICKBED AND RESTORES THEM FROM THEIR BED OF ILLNESS.

PSALM 41: 3

What a beautiful reminder of God's faithfulness and care for us even in our weak moments. No matter what struggles we face, his love and grace never fail. It's in those moments of vulnerability and hardship that we can truly experience the depth of his unfailing love and unwavering support.

When we feel overwhelmed and weary, we can find solace in knowing that God is always by our side, ready to uplift and strengthen us. His faithfulness is like a guiding light in the darkness, leading us towards hope and renewal. Let us take comfort in the knowledge that we are never alone, for God's love surrounds us always, offering comfort, peace, and unwavering support.

_____
_____
_____
_____
_____
_____
_____
_____

Visual Journal

Date: _____

Read the prompts below and respond by filling each space provided with images and words that come into mind.

| When I woke up this morning, I felt..... | Things I wish I can change about today: |

| I am proud of myself today because... | What I prayed for today.... |

Pay Attention - Day 24

MY SON, PAY ATTENTION TO WHAT I SAY; TURN YOUR EAR TO MY WORDS.
DO NOT LET THEM OUT OF YOUR SIGHT,
KEEP THEM WITHIN YOUR HEART;
FOR THEY ARE LIFE TO THOSE WHO FIND THEM AND HEALTH TO ONE'S WHOLE BODY.
PROVERBS 4: 20-22

Just imagine if we took God's words like we take medication to help our illnesses. Just like how we carefully follow the instructions on a prescription bottle, we can also adhere to the teachings and guidance found in His words. The beauty of this metaphor is that, much like adjusting a medication dosage under the supervision of a doctor, we can adjust the doses of God's words as many times as we need to without overdoing it. This flexibility allows us to tailor our spiritual nourishment to our unique needs and circumstances, helping us grow in faith and find strength in times of trouble. So let us approach God's words with the same seriousness and commitment as we do with our health, knowing that they have the power to heal our bodies, our hearts, and uplift our souls.

_____
_____
_____
_____
_____
_____
_____
_____

Visual Journal

Date: _____

Read the prompts below and respond by filling each space provided with images and words that come into mind.

| When I woke up this morning, I felt..... | Things I wish I can change about today: |

| I am proud of myself today because... | What I prayed for today.... |

Worship – Day 25

WORSHIP THE LORD YOUR GOD, AND HIS BLESSING WILL BE ON YOUR FOOD AND WATER. I WILL TAKE AWAY SICKNESS FROM AMONG YOU
EXODUS 23: 25

There is healing in worship! Worship the LORD your God with all your heart and soul, and His blessings will overflow in every aspect of your life. When you honor Him and follow His commandments, He promises to bestow His favor upon you. As it is written, "Worship the LORD your God, and his blessing will be on your food and water. I will take away sickness from among you." This gives us the hope and assurance that God is our healer and protector. Trust in His promises and have faith that He will take away all sickness and bless you abundantly. Let us continuously seek the presence of the Lord and receive His bountiful blessings in our lives.

_____
_____
_____
_____
_____
_____
_____
_____

Visual Journal

Date: _____

Read the prompts below and respond by filling each space provided with images and words that come into mind.

When I woke up this morning, I felt.....	Things I wish I can change about today:
I am proud of myself today because...	What I prayed for today....

Serve - Day 26

SHARE YOUR FOOD WITH THE HUNGRY AND OPEN YOUR HOMES TO THE HOMELESS POOR. GIVE CLOTHES TO THOSE WHO HAVE NOTHING TO WEAR, AND DO NOT REFUSE TO HELP YOUR OWN RELATIVES. THEN MY FAVOR WILL SHINE ON YOU LIKE THE MORNING SUN, AND YOUR WOUNDS WILL BE QUICKLY HEALED.
ISAIAH 58: 7-8

By extending a helping hand to your own relatives and those less fortunate, you are demonstrating love and empathy. In return, you may find blessings and healing in your own life. Just as the morning sun brings warmth and light, your acts of kindness can bring hope and positivity to others and to yourself. Pray about areas where you can help others and list them below. Check them off one by one!

_____
_____
_____
_____
_____
_____
_____

Visual Journal

Date: _____

Read the prompts below and respond by filling each space provided with images and words that come into mind.

| When I woke up this morning, I felt..... | Things I wish I can change about today: |

| I am proud of myself today because... | What I prayed for today.... |

Kind Words - Day 27

PLEASANT WORDS ARE AS AN HONEYCOMB, SWEET TO THE SOUL, AND HEALTH TO THE BONES.
PROVERBS 16: 24

Pleasant words are like a soothing balm for the soul, offering healing to the deepest parts of our being. Just like a honeycomb dripping with sweet nectar, kind and uplifting words have the power to nourish and strengthen us. They provide a sense of warmth and joy that can uplift our spirits and bring light to even the darkest of days. Let us remember the profound impact that our words can have on others, and strive to spread positivity and encouragement wherever we go. In a world that can often feel harsh and unforgiving, let us be beacons of light and hope through the simple but powerful act of speaking kindly and compassionately. Make a list of every person that you said a kind word to today, then pray for them.

_____
_____
_____
_____
_____
_____
_____
_____

Visual Journal

Date: _____

Read the prompts below and respond by filling each space provided with images and words that come into mind.

When I woke up this morning, I felt.....	Things I wish I can change about today:
I am proud of myself today because...	What I prayed for today....

He Still Heals - Day 28

JESUS SAW THE HUGE CROWD AS HE STEPPED FROM THE BOAT, AND HE HAD COMPASSION ON THEM AND HEALED THEIR SICK. MATTHEW 14:14

The Lord, in His infinite grace and compassion, never fails to show His mercy towards the suffering of His people. In times of hardship and distress, He is always there! Through His boundless love, He provides strength and hope to the downtrodden, guiding them through the worst of times. His mercy knows no bounds, reaching out to all who call upon His name with sincerity and faith. Invite Him into your heart and your home so that He will display that same compassion.

Write down your prayer and give it to Him.

_____
_____
_____
_____
_____
_____
_____
_____

Visual Journal

Date: _____

Read the prompts below and respond by filling each space provided with images and words that come into mind.

When I woke up this morning, I felt.....	Things I wish I can change about today:
I am proud of myself today because...	What I prayed for today....

Trust in the Lord – Day 29

TRUST IN THE LORD WITH ALL YOUR HEART AND LEAN NOT ON YOUR OWN UNDERSTANDING; IN ALL YOUR WAYS SUBMIT TO HIM, AND HE WILL MAKE YOUR PATHS STRAIGHT.
DO NOT BE WISE IN YOUR OWN EYES; FEAR THE LORD AND SHUN EVIL.
THIS WILL BRING HEALTH TO YOUR BODY
AND NOURISHMENT TO YOUR BONES. PROVERBS 3: 5-8

Since we know that He is fully powerful, fully present, fully aware, and fully concerned, we should trust Him with all our hearts, even when it requires abandoning our own understanding. In moments of doubt or uncertainty, it is essential to remind ourselves of His infinite wisdom and love. By surrendering our need for control and embracing faith in His plans, we can find peace and clarity in even the most challenging situations. Letting go of our preconceived notions and trusting in his divine guidance can lead us down paths we never imagined possible. So, with unwavering belief and unwavering trust, we can navigate life's twists and turns knowing that we are in His capable hands. What are you letting go of today?

_____
_____
_____
_____
_____
_____
_____
_____

Visual Journal

Date: _____

Read the prompts below and respond by filling each space provided with images and words that come into mind.

When I woke up this morning, I felt.....	Things I wish I can change about today:
I am proud of myself today because...	What I prayed for today....

Safe in His Arms - Day 30

THE LORD IS MY SHEPHERD, I LACK NOTHING. HE MAKES ME LIE DOWN IN GREEN PASTURES, HE LEADS ME BESIDE QUIET WATERS, HE REFRESHES MY SOUL. HE GUIDES ME ALONG THE RIGHT PATHS FOR HIS NAME'S SAKE. EVEN THOUGH I WALK THROUGH THE DARKEST VALLEY, I WILL FEAR NO EVIL, FOR YOU ARE WITH ME; YOUR ROD AND YOUR STAFF, THEY COMFORT ME. YOU PREPARE A TABLE BEFORE ME IN THE PRESENCE OF MY ENEMIES. YOU ANOINT MY HEAD WITH OIL; MY CUP OVERFLOWS. SURELY YOUR GOODNESS AND LOVE WILL FOLLOW ME ALL THE DAYS OF MY LIFE, AND I WILL DWELL IN THE HOUSE OF THE LORD FOREVER. PSALM 23

Psalm 23 beautifully articulates the profound message of God's grace and guidance in our lives. It serves as a poignant reminder that we need not succumb to fear in the face of evil, for God is our protector and shield. This passage reassures us of His unwavering presence and care, urging us to trust in His divine providence. Through the words of Psalm 23, we are reminded of God's abundant blessings and provisions that He graciously bestows upon us, showering His love and mercy upon His faithful followers. As we meditate on these timeless verses, we find comfort in the assurance that God's sovereign reign encompasses all aspects of our lives, leading us in paths of righteousness and peace.

_____
_____
_____
_____
_____
_____
_____
_____

Visual Journal

Date: _____

Read the prompts below and respond by filling each space provided with images and words that come into mind.

When I woke up this morning, I felt.....	Things I wish I can change about today:

I am proud of myself today because...	What I prayed for today....

Notes

Notes

Notes

Notes

Notes

Notes

About the Author

Michelle is a courageous breast cancer survivor who has overcome numerous challenges with unwavering faith. She was diagnosed with breast cancer the same month the world shut down due to Covid-19; through her journey, she rediscovered the power of prayer and its ability to bring comfort and strength during difficult times.

Inspired by her own experiences, Michelle has created a unique prayer journal filled with 30 heartfelt prayers that offer strength and hope to those facing adversity. With a heart full of gratitude and a desire to support others on their spiritual path, Michelle's passion for sharing her story and uplifting words shines through in every page of this journal.

Michelle is also a minister of the Gospel of Jesus Christ, serving in ministry for over two decades and is a current partner at New Foundation Church International, under the leadership of Apostle Sam and Dr. Rico Wagner.

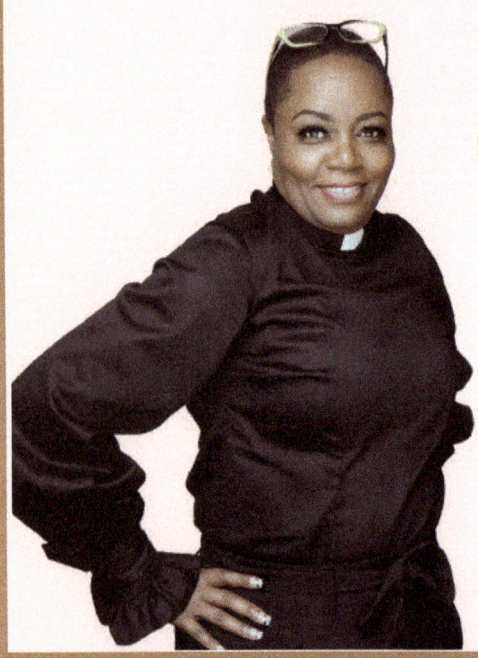

Michelle is a devoted wife to her husband Dexter and a loving mother to four daughters: Emani, Eyanna, Sh'Kee, and D'Zhae; her nephew, Racheon; two granddaughters, Kylar and Clover; one grandson, Amir, and nieces, Olivia, Nova and Ava. She considers herself a God-given mother to many sons and daughters, providing love, guidance, and support to all those around her. With a compassionate heart and nurturing spirit, Michelle's life is centered around her family and creating a warm and loving home for all. Her dedication to her loved ones "shinez" through in everything she does, and she is truly cherished by all who know her.

www.ingramcontent.com/pod-product-compliance
Lightning Source LLC
LaVergne TN
LVHW072120060526
838201LV00068B/4929